THIS IS NOT A DRILL

BREATHE

A Little Book to Help You Prepare for Battle
If You Contract COVID-19

Richard Fenker, PhD

This book offers information on breathing and related topics, but the content is not intended to be a substitute for professional medical or psychological advice, diagnosis, or treatment. The author is not providing healthcare, mental healthcare, medical services, or attempting to diagnose, treat, prevent, or cure in any manner whatsoever any physical ailment, or any mental or emotional issue, disease, or condition. Learning to breathe well supports good health but always seek the advice of your physician or other qualified health provider with any questions you may have regarding the medical conditions associated with COVID-19 or breathing as described in this book and the related treatments.

978-0-9894600-4-6 (paperback)

978-0-9894600-5-3 (ebook)

Published by Cimarron International Publishing
865A Camino Los Abuelos
Galisteo, NM 87540

(505) 820-1686

rich@richardfenker.com

Vector graphics derived from Freepik

For Logan—a constant reminder that DEATH is always nearby, waiting patiently, on my shoulder.

Time is Precious

Time is precious because you and I and millions of others on this planet, in this lifetime, may have little of it left to spend. Let's not waste a second.

At the moment, only a small percentage of people on the Earth currently have COVID-19. But there is a good chance that you or me or our family or our friends will catch the virus this year or in the next few years. Most will have light to moderate symptoms and be able to recover at home, but many will need to go to the hospital.

You have seen the images on TV. They are terrifying. If you enter the hospital with the coronavirus, you are likely to be frightened, isolated from your family, and surrounded by brave healthcare personnel wearing masks and gowns who are also afraid.

Regardless of whether you are currently engaged in social distancing and doing your best to avoid COVID-19, have a mild version of the virus and are recuperating at home or are in the hospital fighting the virus, you need to be ready for the battle of your life.

This little book is designed to help prepare you for this battle and to connect you to those you love and those who will care for you, if you do get to the hospital.

To win this battle only one thing matters --- you must continue to BREATHE.

Now I lay me down to sleep,

I pray the Lord my soul to keep;

If I should die before I wake,

I pray the Lord my soul to take.

Author's Note

For most of my life breathing normally has been both a challenge and a blessing. I suffered from seasonal allergies or hay fever growing up, in part because dad was a smoker. When I was tested for allergies in college it turned out I had a strong reaction not just to smoke but to every grass, every tree and most other things in the kit they used. A short time later, a shot with a tiny amount of allergen given as part of my desensitization treatment produced such a strong response that I could not breathe and turned blue until rescued by the physicians.

Nasal sprays and antihistamines were common remedies that brought some relief, but my breathing was always restricted. When allergies were bad, I was also frequently on the edge of being asthmatic, with the shift from inhaling normally to wheezing close by. My solution was to fight this by grabbing anxiously for air and to breathe faster and harder. Often this resulted in a shot of fear --- that I would not have enough air --- followed by adrenalin and still more desperate breathing.

When I started teaching psychology at TCU in 1968, I became interested in meditation and relaxation techniques, both of which focused on the breath. I soon learned that if (when I was short of breath) I stopped fighting anxiously for air and instead relaxed and breathed more calmly and deeply, allowing the air to fill my lungs --- all of the oxygen I needed was present. Soon, when my allergies were bad, I found all of the breath that was needed without pushing the edges of asthma. Thankfully, this has continued until today.

This little book was written as a reminder to me and to others that when times are tough, breathing "better" is much more important than breathing "harder." And, if you can add good, healthy thoughts to this process that provide positive direction and support this will also help.

Richard Fenker

Contents

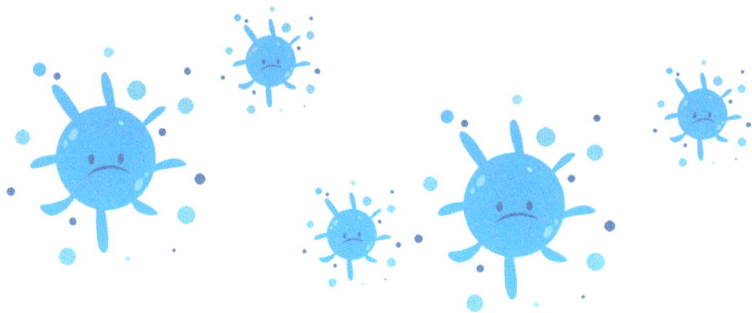

INTRODUCTION:
The Battle for Your Life

In the blink of an eye we have skipped from "flu season" into a full-scale, global battle that will prove deadlier than all the past century's wars combined. If you have been on the sidelines, self-quarantined at home, watching the drama unfold on TV, you may not realize how deadly and dangerous COVID-19 is or how likely it is that much of the world's population will eventually contract it.

Although a virus is not considered to be "living" by most scientists, it comes "alive" by replication once it comes in contact with human cells. COVID-19 is especially dangerous and highly deadly because of the ease of transmission, the lack of symptoms in many cases, and its vicious attacks on a compromised respiratory system or other bodily systems such as the heart or kidneys. I sincerely hope that you and I and most others never contract the virus. But this is certainly not guaranteed, no matter how carefully we behave.

Sadly, many humans on this planet are or soon will be in a battle for their lives. While most will not die, the number who will is staggering.

We are under attack. It's time to fight back by preparing ourselves.

It is All About the Breath

COVID-19, like a seasonal respiratory flu, impacts your body in many ways, but, ultimately, in the end, it deprives you of the oxygen you need to live. Breathing devices, oxygen tanks, respirators, ventilators, medicines, and other aids can help. Fortunately, most people with these medicines, tools or temporary mechanical support will live and breathe normally again.

However, anything helpful you can do now, before you contract the virus, if you contract it with a mild version, or if you are hospitalized, may save your life.

Most creatures on the Earth, including the Earth itself, breathe to support and nourish life. Breathing for everyone, on land or in the ocean, involves finding a delicate balance between the oxygen and carbon dioxide needed. In humans, the virus attacks our respiratory system directly by restricting access to oxygen or indirectly through other diseases such as asthma, heart disease or pneumonia.

Preparing for COVID-19 means doing everything we can NOW to improve our breathing. PART 1 of the book describes six things you can do to help your breath.

Reach Out to Those You Love Now

The stages of development with this virus can go very quickly from benign to serious and chaotic to deadly in the blink of an eye. You may not have time to prepare once you are diagnosed with COVID-19, so you need to prepare now.

Nourishing the breath is part of this preparation. The other part is about nourishing your heart. If you have to fight the coronavirus you will need the strength that comes from the energy, support and love that the people who care for you will have to share. With a mild case of the virus you will be at home and receiving love and support from family and others. But if you are hospitalized, things can change quickly, and you may be alone with loved ones denied access. Now is the time to receive their love and to your share your own thoughts, while you are healthy, before the battle begins --- just in case.

Think of this effort as you might think of creating your will or medical directives. It is a way of quickly giving and receiving love by documenting your thoughts.

Last but not least we don't want to forget the physicians, nurses, emergency staff and others who may end up caring for you. They also need your love and thanks.

PART 2 of the book offers three brief exercises to help you build these important connections.

PART 3 presents information on four different breathing techniques designed to help you breathe in a more relaxed, effective manner when you are under stress.

PART 1:
The Breath

Here are six key techniques to help enhance your breathing:

Make Your Self-Talk an Ally

Let Go of Fear

Use the Power of Your Imagination

Embrace Death

Listen to Your Spirit

Nourish the Breath

SPEAK FROM THE HEART: Make Your Self-Talk an Ally

The constant talking voice in your head, known as self-talk, is largely responsible for the reality that you experience in every moment.

Self-talk is a mix of factual content—*this stone wall is hard, or the sun is bright today*—and opinions based on your beliefs, your education, your family, your work, and many other influences. Some of these opinions may be factually correct—*physicians are generally good, caring people*—but most are a mixture of fact and fiction. Think of them as beliefs that you have adopted as part of your unique version of reality.

What is important about self-talk is that **the words you speak to yourself determine, to a large degree, how you feel and how you will behave in most circumstances**. Happy, positive words often lead to good outcomes experienced in a pleasant, supportive world. Negative, angry words often create stress and experiences that are more likely to be perceived as unhappy and non-supportive.

The actual, real world is neutral. Your reality can be hot or cold, friendly or hostile, supportive or not, based on your self-talk.

To prepare for a battle with the coronavirus, you need self-talk that is positive, supportive, and sends your mind and body in the best directions to stay healthy and nourish your breath.

Affirmations are a simple but powerful tool to do this.

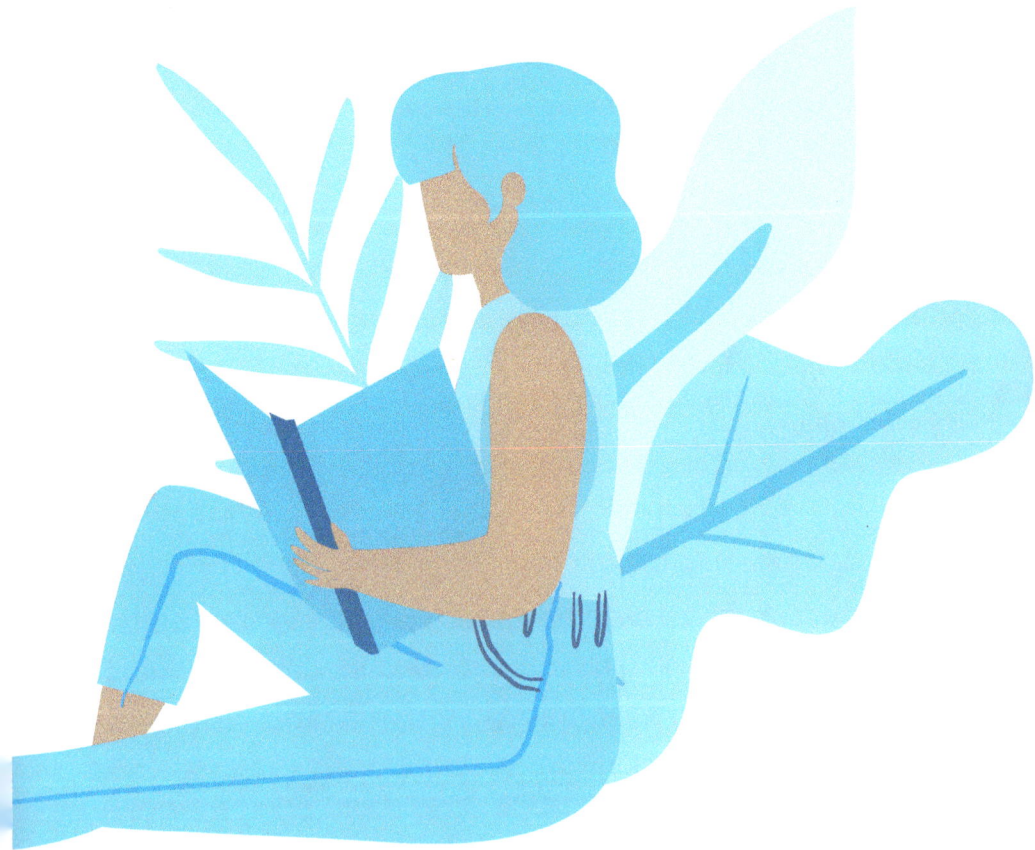

An affirmation is a short, positive statement that you repeat to yourself as a way of focusing your self-talk in the directions you want. Affirmations replace negative thoughts and ruminations that are stressful and compromise breathing. Here are a couple of examples:

My mind and body are strong and capable.
My immune system is a mighty fortress
that will protect me against the coronavirus.
It will fight to block the virus from entering my body
or destroy it, if it penetrates these defenses.

OR

I am not alone.
I am part of a world filled with oxygen
and help to support my breathing.
When I feel a shortness of breath,
instead of fighting and breathing harder,
I will relax and breathe more deeply,
pulling cool, rich air from the world around me
into my lungs.

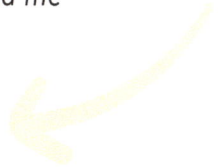

These are only examples. Go to the internet, type "affirmations for health" or "affirmations for breathing" into the search box and you will be overwhelmed with examples of self-talk you can use that best fits your personal needs.

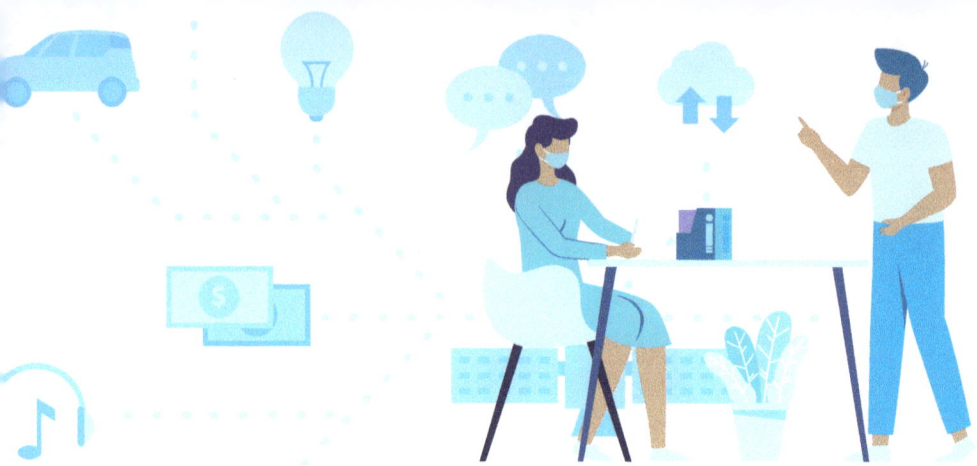

FEAR: Let Go of Your Fear

COVID-19 and the resulting global pandemic it has created is terrifying. Watching the news each day, remaining in isolation—and on occasional trips into the world, seeing the masks everywhere and fear in the eyes of store clerks, bus drivers, healthcare workers and others who cannot isolate themselves—is frightening. And it is difficult not to let this fear become part of our everyday self-talk.

Yet fear, like stress and our body's emergency "fight or flight" response, are all mechanisms that, while helpful when needed, are also deadly when activated constantly over a long period of time. Why? Because they sap the body's energy and reserve strength needed to fight disease.

Also, while all these mechanisms temporarily increase oxygen in your system by increasing your respiration rate, this extra effort to breathe faster interferes with the normal, relaxed breathing processes needed to maintain your health in an emergency.

Changing fearful self-talk to positive self-talk and learning to let go of the fear with your breathing are key survival skills that will help if you contract the virus.

First, interrupt the fearful self-talk with a simple, positive affirmation.

> *I choose not to be afraid.*
> *I acknowledge my fearful thoughts but then let go of them.*
> *With each exhalation I release some of these thoughts*
> *from inside my body to the atmosphere around me,*
> *where they will disappear.*
> *I am strong and healthy.*
> *I am filled with confidence and courage.*

Then, shift your mind to your breathing. Notice your current breaths for a moment. Perhaps they are shallow and quick. Perhaps not. Now, take a deep breath and feel your lungs expand. Hold the air for a few seconds and then exhale, imaging yourself releasing some of the fear and stress into the space around you as you breathe out.

After a few breaths repeat the affirmation above or one that you create for yourself. This cycle—affirmation / focus on your breathing / affirmation—will interrupt the fearful thoughts and allow your self-talk to shift to positive, healthy words.

Remember, what you say to yourself creates much of the reality that you experience!

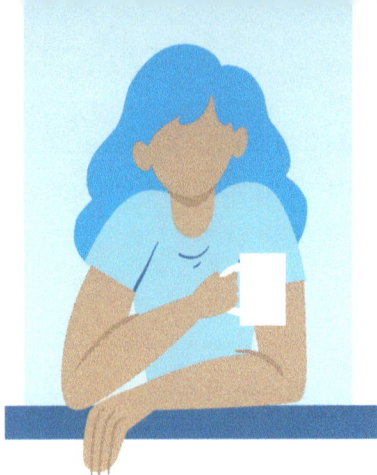

IMAGINE: Create a Vision for Your Listening Mind

While conversations coming from the talking mind are likely to dominate your day, working in the background (and just as important) is a quiet mind. Think of it as the listening mind that is the target of the talker's conversations.

While the talking mind is caught up in words and logic and sequences, the listening mind is more attached to images or concepts or whole things. For example, the talking mind sees a golf swing as a sequence of steps. Take the club back, break your wrists, and so on. The listening mind or quiet mind sees a holistic image or picture of the entire swing.

Notice that to swing a golf club, hit a home run, kick a soccer ball, or do most other physical activities YOU DO NOT NEED TO THINK OF THE SEQUENCE OF STEPS REQUIRED. The quiet, visual mind has you covered! These are all well-rehearsed patterns that it remembers and can use automatically. If someone tosses you a ball, you don't think about how to catch it, you just reach out and catch.

Your quiet mind is a major ally for your health. Just as it remembers, automatically, how to catch a ball, it also knows what it is like to have a completely healthy body and mind. If your vision of yourself is that "you are a tower of energy and health," your quiet mind will be constantly executing this vision in the world.

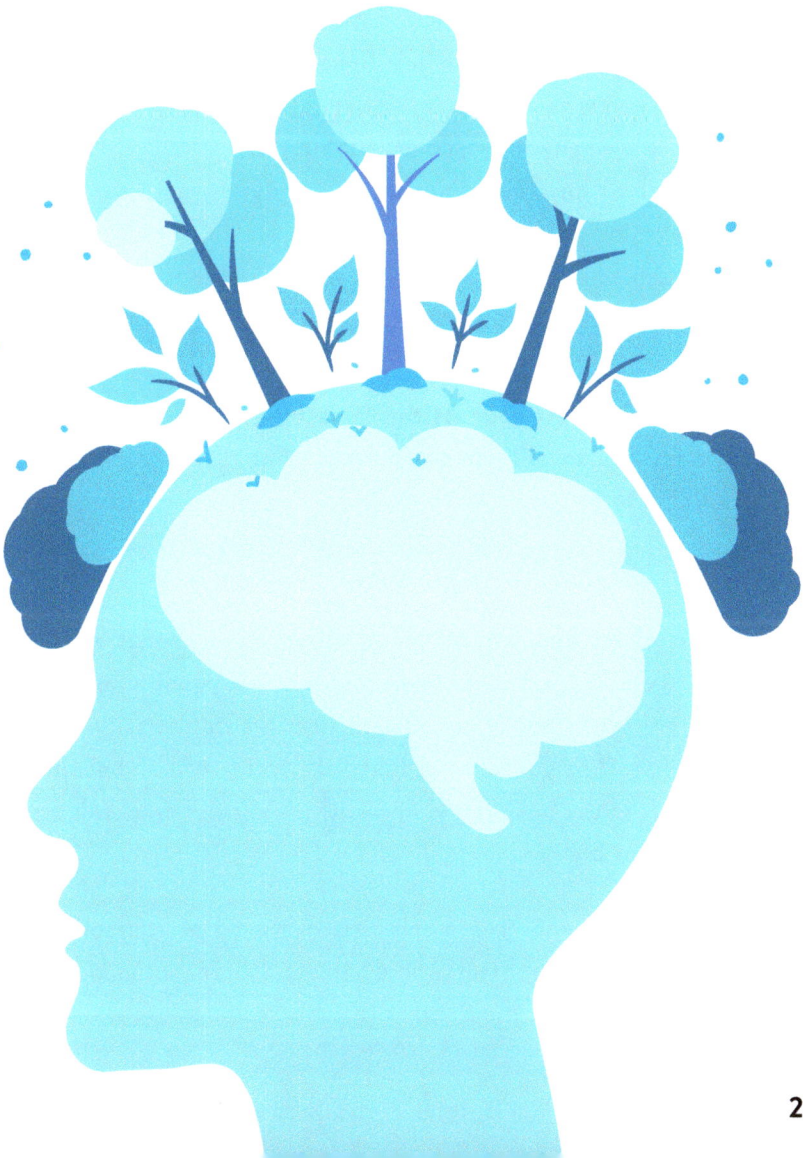

To prepare for the coronavirus and to defeat it with your overwhelming healthiness, we need the quiet mind on your side. We need for it to have a clear vision of you and your immune system as healthy and strong and capable of blocking or minimizing any disease—just like the golf swing—so that it can execute this image perfectly, over and over, automatically, without any conscious effort on your part.

We need the quiet mind, in the background, supporting all the systems in your body that underlie healthy breathing. You want it to help fight a lack of enough oxygen with relaxation, not agitation and gasping, knowing that left alone, without the fear coming from conscious thought, your body and the quiet mind will find a way to give you all of the air you need. And if this is not possible, to let your physicians know.

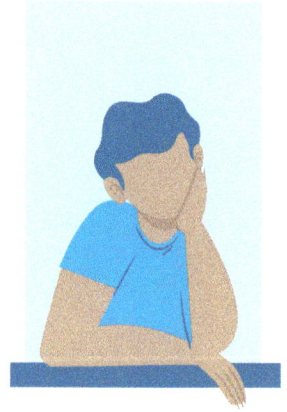

We used words to create your affirmations. Now let's use an image to tell the quiet mind what you would like to happen.

Imagine yourself as healthy and strong—so strong that any illness, even COVID-19, is just an inconvenience that your immune system and other healthy bodily systems will handle automatically, minimizing its impact, so you will not feel sick. And if you do become sick at home or in the hospital, your healthy body and mind will protect you and your breath.

Take a moment and create this healthy vision of yourself in your mind; then remind yourself of it when you feel fear or anxiety about the virus. Your quiet mind wants to protect you and it will.

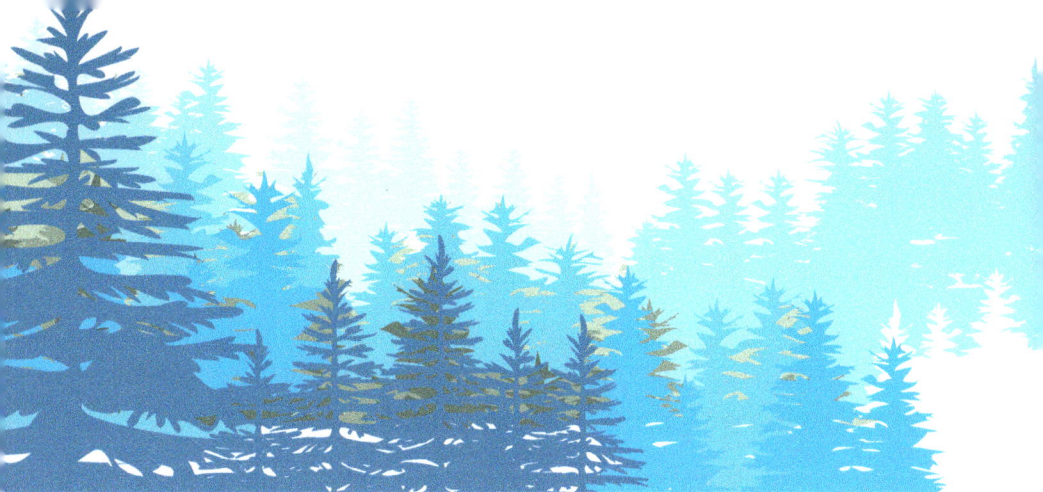

DEATH: Embrace Death to Defuse Its Power

What is unique about the coronavirus, compared with most diseases, is that it is a relentless killer. It attacks the weak. It finds those with weak respiratory systems and other vulnerable areas and then, launches a merciless assault. Conversations and statistics about the virus are often conversations about death because the threat of death is real for anyone who catches the virus, especially the elderly.

What makes this especially difficult for most cultures is that death is a taboo subject to be avoided. We don't talk about death. We get to the edges of a conversation about death with medical directives and wills and long-term care options, but generally, we live in denial. This is what makes the death statistics from the virus so terrifying.

Much of death's power over us comes from this denial. By defining death-related conversations as inappropriate or uncomfortable we end up avoiding the topic, making death the omnipresent "elephant in the room." How would you feel if your spouse or father or best friend or child went to the hospital with COVID-19 and never returned? And, what if you missed the opportunity to say goodbye or share in rituals that would typically be part of a good death?

What if it was you going to the hospital, alone and scared and without the opportunity to discuss your possible death and the consequences of your death with your family?

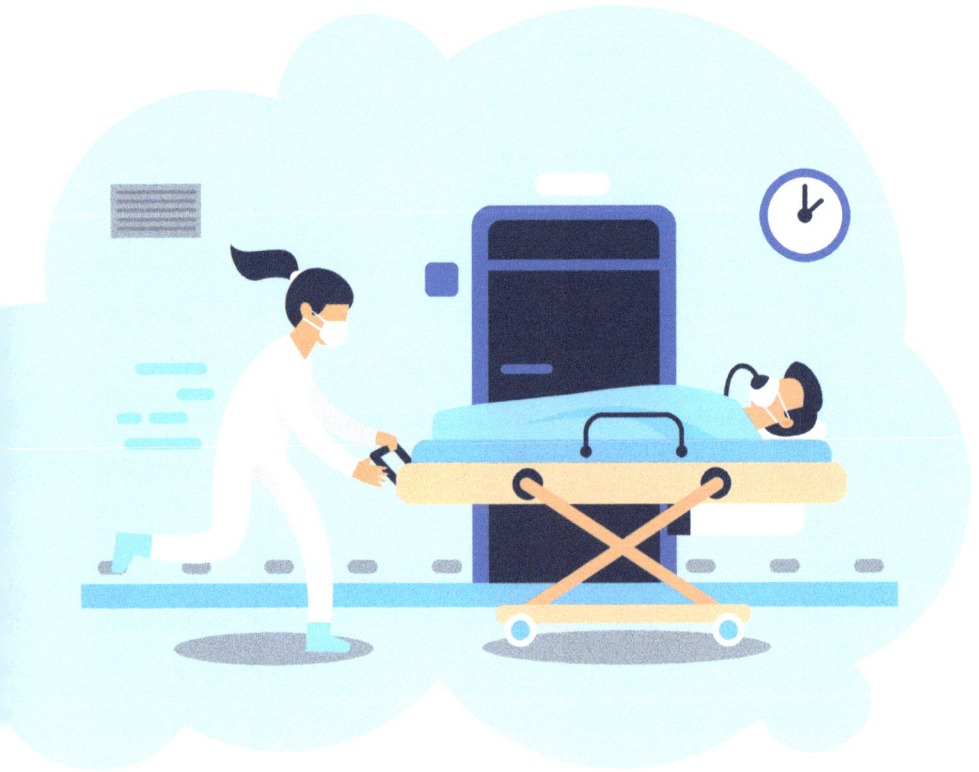

You and I, of course, will eventually die. Let's hope it is not from COVID-19. But instead of running from this fact and retreating into more comfortable areas for a conversation, if we embrace death, an amazing thing happens. Our death becomes, in our self-talk, what it represents in reality, just another normal event. It's OK to talk about it, plan around it, tease or joke about it and so forth. In the open it is just another part of our reality. In the dark it can be the source of much fear and anxiety.

To demystify death and steal its power, there are three brief things I want you to do as soon as you finish reading the book:

1. CREATE A LEGACY: What would you like your children, grandchildren or others in the future to know about you? Write 4-5 bullet points that represent a brief legacy that describes how you would like to be remembered by future generations.

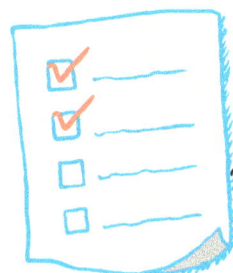

2. MAKE A PLAN TO LIVE FULLY NOW: If you knew that you only had one year to live, what would you do during this year? Write 4-5 bullet points that describe your plans. Perhaps these are items on your "bucket list." Perhaps they represent changes in what you do every day or things you would like to share with those close to you. Perhaps you are already doing some of these things. It doesn't matter. What is important is that your list pushes you not to wait but to live more fully now.

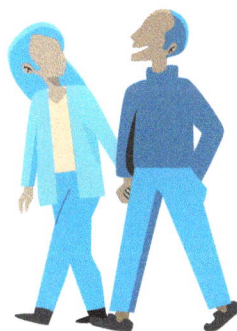

3. WRITE A FIVE-MINUTE OBIT: Contrary to our common beliefs, you don't need to be dead to have an obituary! A good obit is both a brief statement of how you would like to be remembered (when you are dead) and how you would like to be perceived now by the family and friends you care most about. To be remembered as caring or generous or adventurous, for example, you have to live in this manner today. So, in making a statement about what you want others to say about you after death, you are actually describing how you want to live your current life. Write 4-5 brief bullet points that will be included in your obit and then get to work living these now!

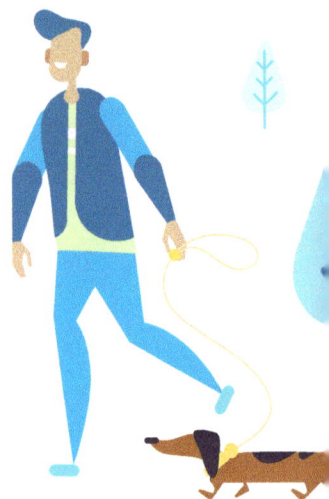

Each of these tasks helps to defuse the energy that death has to make us fearful. Now, if you do battle with COVID-19, your focus can be on staying positive, keeping a healthy image in mind, and breathing.

SPIRIT:
Listen to Your Spirit

The talking mind, the listening mind, our body, breath and all of the other components that make up our physical being, especially our immune system, are warriors in our battle against the coronavirus. But there is another fighter in our corner, so powerful and so full of magic that its light makes all others dim by comparison.

Our spiritual being touches all life on this planet and beyond. Our consciousness lives within Earth's consciousness that gives life, takes life, and can heal. Spirit spurs us to seek out higher goals, to have faith, to care for each other and all things in our world. Spirit fill soldiers with courage, healers with wisdom and power and nourishes anyone unafraid to live outside the boundaries of our everyday consciousness.

Many cultures, religions and faith-oriented practices embrace the magic of spirit as part of their beliefs. The history of man on our majestic Earth is filled with examples where spirit, faith, courage, and love triumphed over man's selfish, ego-oriented consciousness and the associated self-talk.

Regardless of your beliefs, your spirit is always present, always waiting to connect with other beings and minds on our planet, and always capable of miracles.

If you end up in a battle for your life against the coronavirus, your spirit will be there to help. It's the extra spark needed to keep your heart beating. It's the quiet comfort and love, in the background, as your body fights to breathe. It's the magic that bonds you with your healers and soothes your transition between this world and the next.

Anyone who works in the presence of death understands the beauty and power of spirit. As you struggle to breathe, know that your spirit is there to offer you the spark of life needed to keep you breathing and, if necessary, to welcome you across death's threshold.

You are and always will be one with the Earth. Your spirit and your body are products of the Earth, which nourishes you at every moment with light and air and water and sustenance.

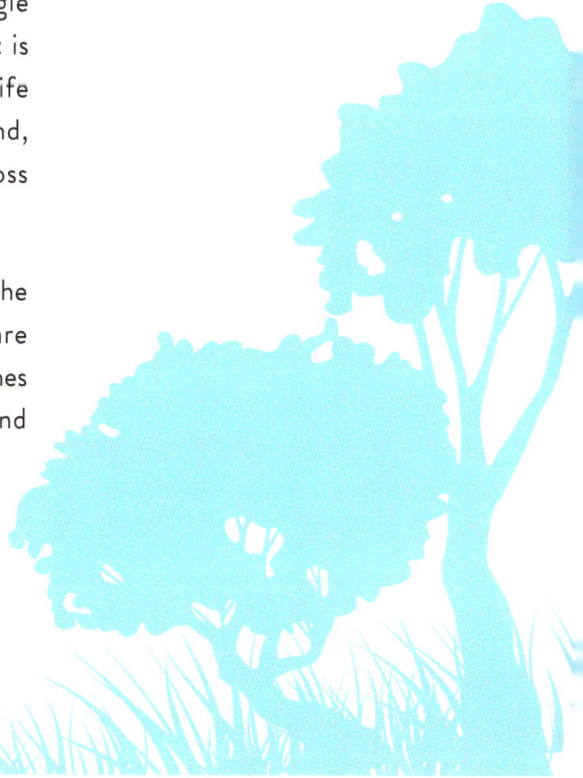

Every breath you take belongs to you and to the Earth. You are not alone. In a moment of crisis, it is there, in the background, to help you breathe.

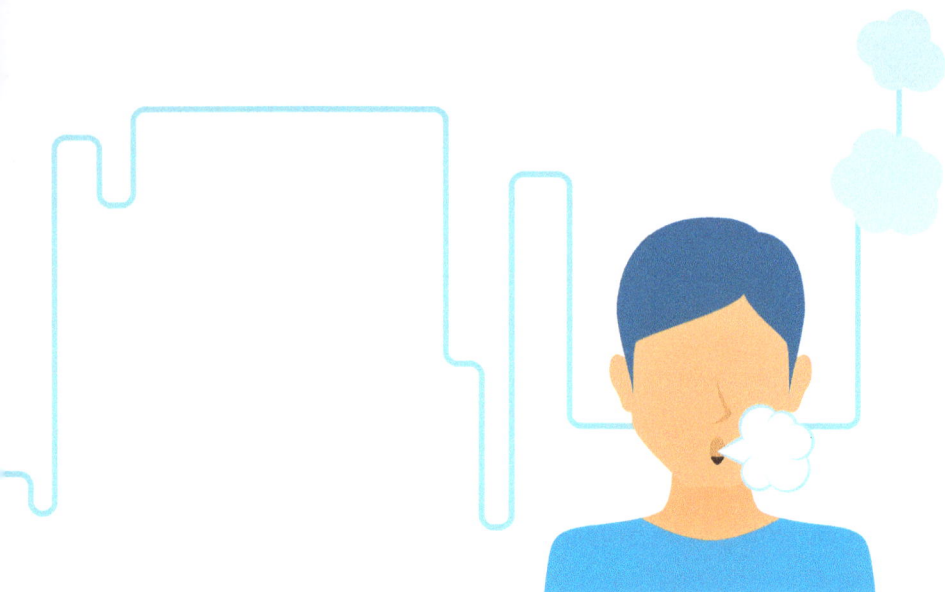

BREATHE: It Is All About the Breath

Defeating COVID-19 is all about breathing. The previous chapters have given you an arsenal of tools to shape the thoughts in your mind, to create a vision of your healthy mind and body, to release fear, to defuse the power of death by embracing it, and much more.

Ultimately, everything comes together in the one single act you need to perform to defeat COVID-19: to breathe, fully and completely.

You can help yourself here, but you are not alone. Breathing deeply, breathing without fear, breathing to nourish your healthy body, breathing air from the edges of the earth, embracing the power of your spirit—all work to keep you healthy and in the fight if the virus attacks your body.

Here is a simple breathing exercise you can use to calm yourself.

AIR: A Breathing Exercise

1. Sit or lie down with your back straight. Inhale deeply and as you exhale, allow your face, neck, jaw, and shoulders to relax. Give a small "sigh" with each exhalation to encourage relaxation.

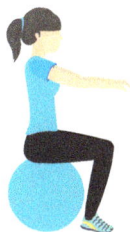

2. Continue breathing and observe your breath for a couple of minutes. Notice the cycle of inhalations and exhalations.

3. Now, as you inhale, feel your chest and ribs and abdomen expand.

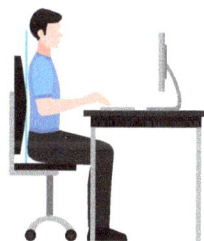

4. Allow any negative thoughts or fears about the virus or breathing or other concerns to sink, momentarily, into your chest.

5. Then, as you exhale, release these concerns and fears out to the universe, feeling the peacefulness inside.

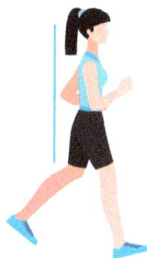

6. Repeat this process 10-15 times. If your mind wanders, that is OK. Gently move your focus back to your breathing.

The first few times you do this exercise you may find yourself distracted and unable to focus. Quickly, however, your body and mind will learn to concentrate, and after a week, you will notice a shift in the intensity and depth of your relaxation.

When you feel fear, shortness of breath, anxiety or tightness in your muscles use this simple exercise to help. Instead of breathing harder and more rapidly, relax and breathe deeply and calmly. All the oxygen you need will be present.

PART 2:
Sharing Love

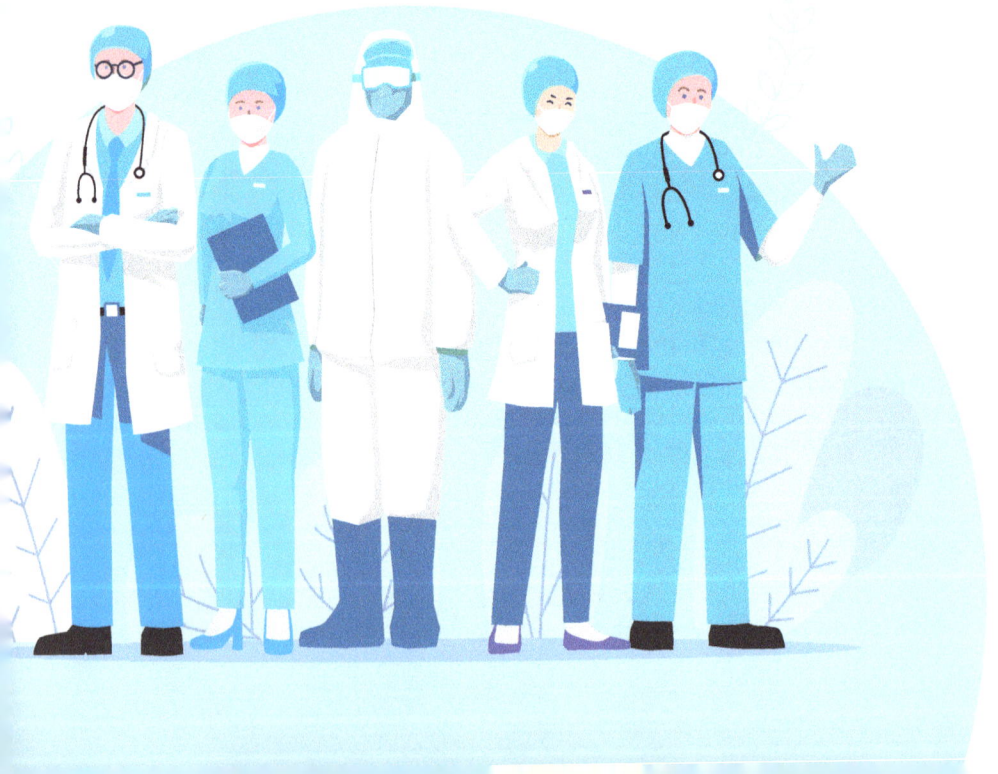

The Three Things You Can Do Now to Share Love

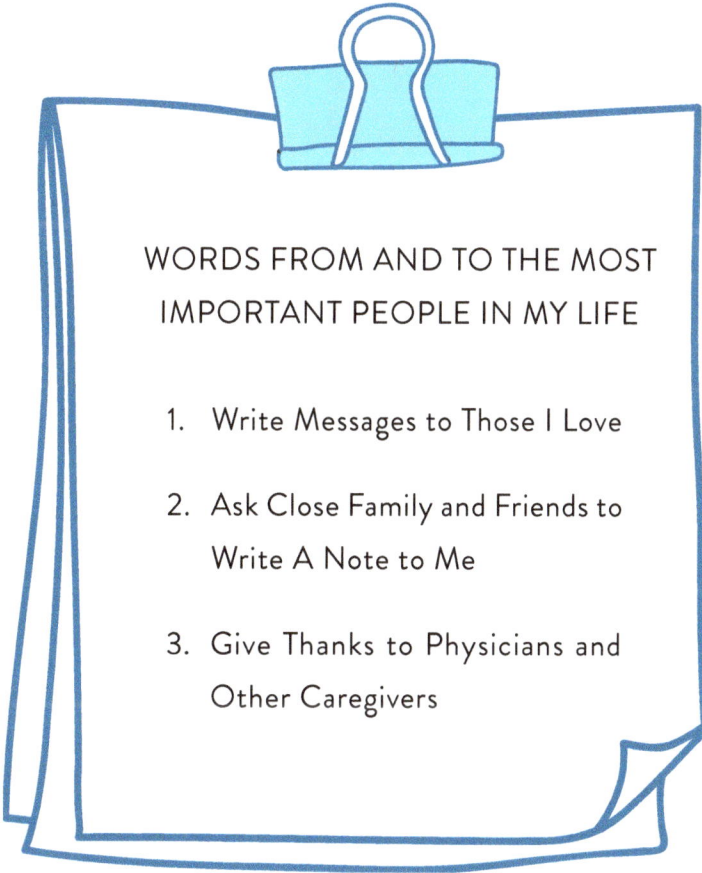

WORDS FROM AND TO THE MOST
IMPORTANT PEOPLE IN MY LIFE

1. Write Messages to Those I Love

2. Ask Close Family and Friends to Write A Note to Me

3. Give Thanks to Physicians and Other Caregivers

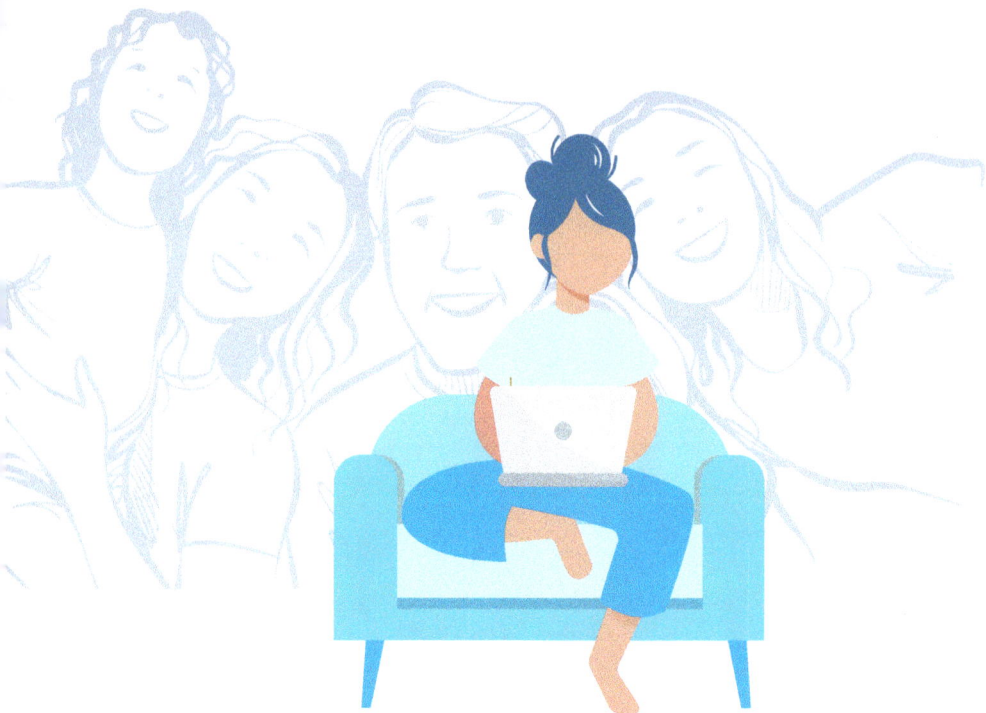

Write Messages to The People You Love

Imagine for a moment that next month will be your last. Let's hope this is not the case! However, because the idea of your death is now something you can plan for, talk about and consider without fear, use this opportunity to share your love. Make your messages to family and friends brief (perhaps just a couple of sentences) and specific. Go for the heart of what you want to say. *"I love you because you have always cared for me in good times and tough times."* Or, *"Your friendship has meant so much to me. You have added a huge amount of joy to my life."*

I realize that you probably have much more to say to these family members and friends; but now is not the time. Tomorrow, next week or next month you can write as much or as little as you want. At the moment the most important thing is to finish all of the exercises in this short book because each different one anchors you in some important way.

Write each message on a separate note card or sheet of paper then you can either share them immediately, share them at a later time or leave them with a friend with instructions to share them if you become ill or go to the hospital. Just writing the messages grounds you in the love you have for others and if things become difficult, these are wonderful thoughts to have in your mind and self-talk.

In critical situations, *regrets* can sap our energy and focus. Finishing this simple exercise means that you will never have to regret that key things your wanted to say to family and friends were lost.

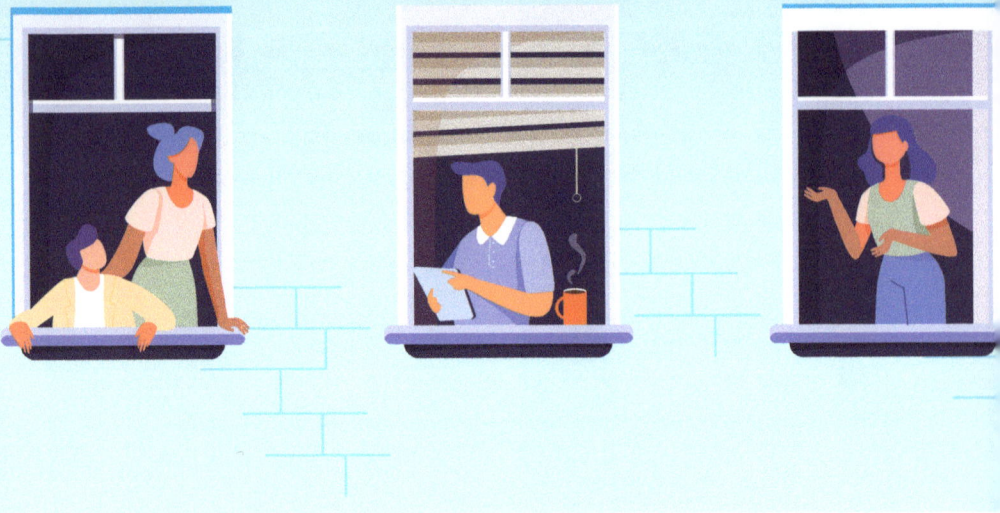

Receive Messages of Love from Family and Friends

Ask the people in your family and the friends that you care about the most to write a short note to you, now, expressing their feelings about you, knowing the note will be opened only if you become very ill or enter the hospital with COVID-19. Tell them to make the messages to you brief, just a sentence or two, and specific. Encourage them to focus on the heart of what they would like to say to you.

"Dear Rich, you have added much joy and inspiration to my life. I am in a different and happier place today thanks to you."

"Dear Rich, you have been a great friend and partner. When I needed help, I could always count on you."

Your family and friends can always choose, at a later time, to write a longer note to you; but, at the moment the key thing is to write a short note quickly and make it available to you. I recommend that you ask one family member to coordinate this activity for you and to keep the notes that people send.

I also think it is fine, if you and your family chose, to open the messages before you have any illness. There is no reason to hold back love.

HEROES:
Cherish the Medical Personnel Who Risk Their Lives to Help

WORDS OF THANKS TO MY CAREGIVERS

THANK YOUR CAREGIVERS: Write a brief thank you note NOW to share with those who will be helping you, if for any reason you need to see a physician or enter the hospital with COVID-19. I've attached a sample note below to give you some ideas. When you finish your note, have it laminated, put into a plastic cover or printed on cloth. Ideally, if you go to the hospital you will be carrying it, wearing it or have it present in some other way so your physicians can see how much you appreciate them.

To my physicians, nurses, and other caregivers.

I love you.

*My heart goes out to you for the courage
you show every day in caring for me.*

I love you because you have risked your own life and wellness,

day after day, to care for me and many others.

*I love you for helping me to breathe,
helping my body to function*

and for keeping me alive while it heals.

*Thank you. I can never repay you for the
kindness you have shown me.*

*May God bless you, your family, and
all others that you care for.*

PART 3:
Keep Breathing

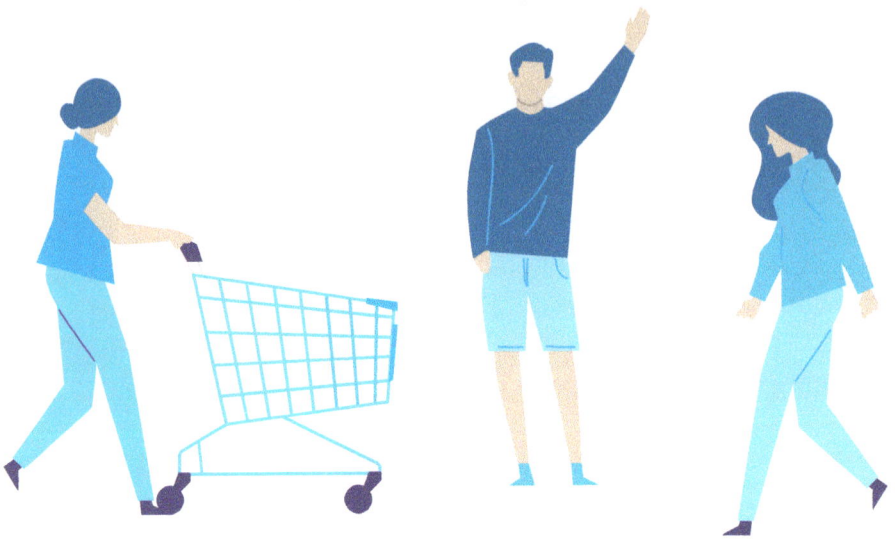

Use A Breathing Exercise to Relax and Reduce Anxiety

You know that relaxing and taking deep breaths is good if you have the coronavirus and want to breathe more effectively. But, how do you do this when you are stressed and fearful? Breathing meditations are a simple but powerful way to use the process of breathing to relax, sleep or essentially "turn off" the talking, fearful mind. The idea is that by focusing your attention on some parts of the process, the noise that your self-talk and anxiety are creating is reduced or eliminated.

This is not a situation where "one size fits all." Breathing is associated with our different senses and each of us uses these in a individual manner. Some of us are very visual (a picture is worth 1,000 words); others are auditory-oriented and sounds have the strongest impact; others depend on words or language --- the voice of a parent or teacher or friend in our mind can be very soothing or instructive. Finally, some of us are kinesthetic or touch oriented. The feeling of our body or our breath is what dominates our senses and responses. The different sensory channels are called sensory modalities. We use all four of the senses or modalities described above but depend most on the dominant one.

Breathing meditations work best when they use our preferred sensory modality. If I give you an exercise for breathing that asks you to visualize your breath coming from across the mountains into your lungs, filling your body with light, this may not work well if you are kinesthetic-oriented and need to concentrate on feeling the breath in your body. For many, exercises that involve counting are natural and effective while for others they can be very distracting. You will need to experiment to discover which approach works best for you. I ended Part 1 of the book with a sample breathing exercise. Perhaps it fits your sensory biases well and is easy to use. Most likely you need some other options to select from to find the best fit.

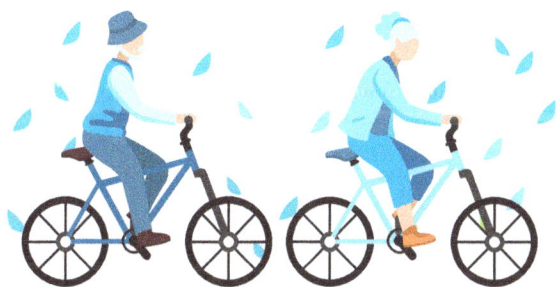

The next section offers four different breathing exercises designed to help you relax and breathe more effectively. Each exercise in some way engages and distracts the talking mind, often the source of much stress, to shift your attention to a healthier place. Dozens of examples of breathing meditations can be found online if none of my examples is optimum for you. Please note that all of these approaches use two or more of your sensory modalities.

Remember that your battle with COVID-19, even when you have excellent care from your physicians and a loving family, is likely to be a lonely one. Every small thing you can do now and later to help breathe better can have a huge influence. The breathing exercises use your mind and your body to provide this help. Even in the darkest of times these tools for breathing belong to you. They are important weapons in your arsenal. You are not helpless. Remind yourself that, regardless of the circumstances, you are in this fight to win.

FOUR BREATHING EXERCISES

1 Breathing and Relaxing the Body (Kinesthetic and Verbal Senses)

▸ Find a comfortable position sitting or lying down.

▸ Take a couple of deep breaths and release the air with a sigh.

▸ Inhale, then hold the breath and tense the muscles in your feet and hands for a few moments.

▸ Now exhale, releasing the tension.

▸ Beginning with your feet, tell them to relax fully and let this relaxed feeling begin to spread gradually upwards to your calves, knees, upper legs and thighs and on into your stomach and chest.

▸ Breathe in and out, allowing this feeling of relaxation to spread into your shoulders and arms and hands.

▸ Now, let these relaxed feelings expand into your neck, your face and finally your scalp.

▸ Your entire body is in a healthy relaxed state. Breathe deeply, in and out, enjoying the feelings of relaxation.

▸ If any part of your body feels tense, focus your mind on it for a second, tighten the muscles and then relax them as you exhale, releasing the tension.

▸ When you have finished relaxing, remain in this relaxed state, breathing deeply, for a few minutes.

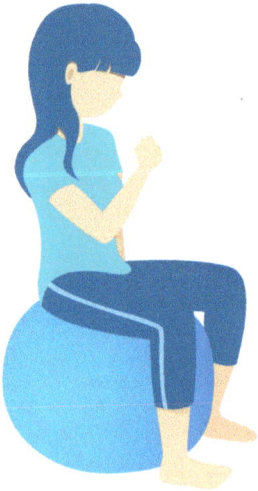

2 Breathing and Counting (Auditory and Kinesthetic Senses)

▶ Find a comfortable position sitting or lying down.

▶ Take a couple of deep breaths and release them with a sigh, emptying the lungs of air.

▶ Breath in through your nose for 3 seconds.

▶ Now hold the breath for 6 seconds.

▶ Finally, purse your lips and exhale through your mouth for 4 seconds with a sigh or whoosh sound.

▶ Repeat this process 3-4 times then return to normal breathing.

▶ Alternate breathing with counting and normal breathing to support relaxation.

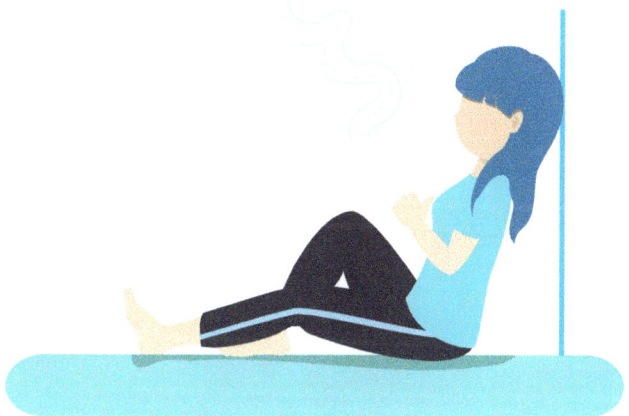

3   Breathing and Feeling the Breath (Visual and Verbal Senses)

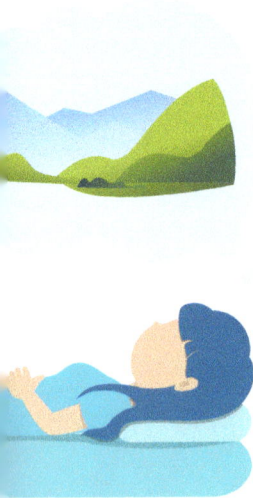

▶ Imagine a beautiful, serene, relaxing place and create the image of this place in your mind. Describe it with a word or phrase. The Padre Island shoreline, where the ocean meets the beach, would be my place and the words *beach shoreline* would describe it to me.

▶ Find a comfortable position sitting or lying down.

▶ Relax, wiggle your shoulders and body releasing any tension, and close your eyes.

▶ Take a few deep breaths releasing each breath with a sigh.

▶ Breathe in deeply, feeling the air bring a sense of peace and calm into your body. Feel your lungs relax and allow the sense of relaxation and calmness to spread throughout the body.

▶ Exhale deeply now and imagine that the breath is pulling the stress and tension and pain from all parts of your body and sending it out into the atmosphere with the air.

▶ As you breathe, imagine that you are in your special place and add words to guide how you want to feel.

▶ For example, with each inhalation you might say to yourself, "I breath in the beauty and serenity of my special place." And then, with each exhalation, "I breathe out all pain and tension."

▶ Each cycle of inhalation and exhalation leaves you calmer and more relaxed.

▶ Repeat this process for 15-20 minutes or until you are calm.

4 Deep Breathing (Kinesthetic Sense)

▶ When the coronavirus challenges our breathing, the result is often short, quick anxious breaths. Slowing down and breathing more deeply reduces fear and tension and increases the air available to our lungs.

▶ Find a comfortable position sitting or lying down. Be sure that your head and shoulders are supported.

▶ Breathe in through your nose and feel the air expand into your lungs and belly. A deep breath can be felt all the way through your stomach.

▶ Now breathe out through your nose, feeling your belly and lungs contract as they empty of air.

▶ Place one hand on your belly and the other on your chest.

▶ As you breathe in and out notice how much your belly rises and sinks. Notice that your chest also moves, but not as much.

▶ Concentrate on your belly rising and falling, moving your hand, as you breathe deeply.

▶ Repeat this process with 4-5 breaths until you feel yourself relax.

▶ With practice your body will learn to quickly relax once you start deep breathing.

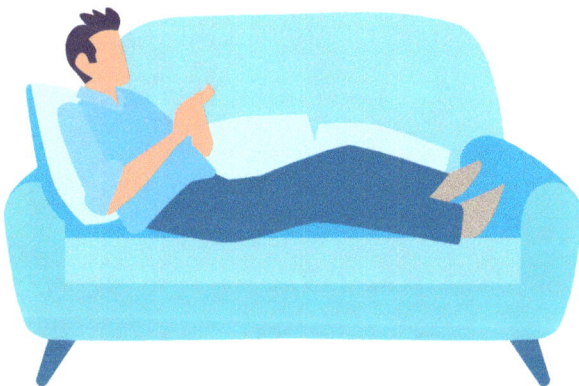

BREATHE: HOW YOU WILL DEFEAT COVID-19

Breathe as if your life depended on it.

Reach out to the universe to pull rich, cool air from its vastness.

Relax and breathe deeply.

Even though you are awake and conscious now, your breathing is automatic and all of the air you need will be available regardless of your condition.

If you are unconscious, your body/mind will still remember to breathe, to bring oxygen and the gift of life to your lungs and body.

You know now to let go of all fear and anxiety to breathe deeply and fully without interference. Your positive affirmations give you the tools to make this happen.

In a moment of crisis, you defeat COVID-19 with your relaxation and trust in the power of your breath. Your body, mind, and spirit are all one and all working together.

This little book is your battle plan. It has gifts to others that will linger long after your death. It has the messages to you that will be part of your deep consciousness forever. It invokes the power of the spirit to heal you and comfort you. And it asks for your forgiveness from the Earth for all the harm we have wrought with our selfishness as humans on this planet.

Now there is only one task left.

To breathe.

Take deep breaths now and at all times.

Help yourself recover by breathing, even in the toughest of situations. On oxygen or a ventilator? Your unconscious mind knows what to do to.

Breathe. Feel the cool, oxygen-rich air enter your lungs bringing life and healing.

Breathe. Know you are surrounded by the love of your family and friends and those working to heal you.

If you experience shortness of breath, fight the coronavirus by relaxing and breathing as deeply as possible. Trust in your body and mind and spirit to find the oxygen you need. Trust in your healers to know when they need to intervene to keep you breathing.

Breathe.

Relax and breathe deeply.

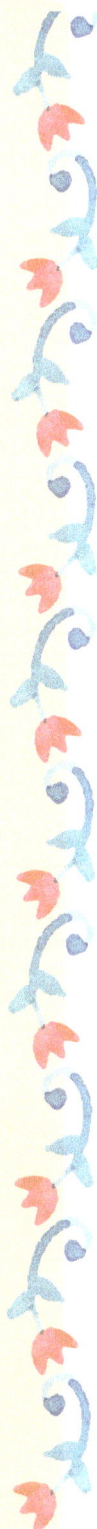

To Those Already Hospitalized with COVID-19

My heart goes out to you. I know this is likely to be a frightening, chaotic, and very stressful time.

You have prepared yourself for battle with the materials in this book.

- You have let the people you love know it and asked for their messages of love to you.

- You have taken away much of death's power to frighten and harm you by making it a normal part of your self-talk.

- You have learned affirmations to reduce your fear and to help strengthen your immune system.

- You have asked your conscious and unconscious minds to work together to create a healthy vision and fight the virus.

- You have learned how to breathe.

Remember that you are not alone. You are surrounded by the love from your family and friends, from the physicians that care for you and from the larger life force that nourishes us all. You are in touch with the magic and power of your spirit, allowing it to give comfort and to heal your body.

Breathe, and in breathing find a way to return to this Earth healthy and healed.

I love your courage and determination and fearlessness.

You are not alone. We are all praying for your safe return.

Richard Fenker

I want to thank the community of kind people, family and friends, who helped with the final editing and proofreading of this little book. This group includes Nancy Reigel, Howard Fenker, Patrick Lane, Cindy Lux, Barbara Holloway, Marilyn Giasson-Fenker and the editor of my previous book, Sandra Wendel, who reviewed an early version and made helpful comments. My cover and book designer, Philadelphia Cardona is responsible for the wonderful, airy design and all of the graphics. Her work really brought the book to life. In creating Breathe I rushed to make it available as quickly as possible and take full responsibility for any errors that you might find.

Richard Fenker is Emeritus Professor of Psychology at Texas Christian University and an author, inventor, and mathematician. He is an expert in human learning, thinking, and consciousness. He is the author of 12 books and several hundred articles in a variety of areas including learning skills, human consciousness, sport psychology, retail site selection, Alzheimer's/dementia, rocket science, mathematics and others.

He currently lives in Santa Fe, New Mexico, with his wife, Marilyn.

www.ingramcontent.com/pod-product-compliance
Lightning Source LLC
Chambersburg PA
CBHW041222030426
42336CB00024B/3419